Revolutionize Your Health:
A Comprehensive Guide to Conquering Type 2 Diabetes Through Diet and Nutrition

Table of Contents:

Chapter 1: Understanding Type 2 Diabetes: The Basics

Type 2 diabetes is a chronic condition that affects millions of people worldwide. It is characterized by high blood sugar levels, which can lead to serious health complications if left untreated. However, with proper management, it is possible to lead a long, healthy life even with this diagnosis. In this chapter, we will cover the basics of Type 2 diabetes, including its causes, symptoms, and diagnosis.

1.1 What is Type 2 Diabetes?

Type 2 diabetes is a metabolic disorder that occurs when the body becomes resistant to insulin, the hormone that regulates blood sugar levels. This leads to high blood sugar levels, which can damage blood vessels, nerves, and organs over time.

1.2 Causes and Risk Factors

Type 2 diabetes is caused by a combination of genetic and lifestyle factors. Some of the most common risk factors include:

* Family history of diabetes

* Being overweight or obese

* Sedentary lifestyle

* Poor diet

* Certain medical conditions, such as polycystic ovary syndrome (PCOS)

1.3 Symptoms and Diagnosis

Symptoms of Type 2 diabetes can include:

* Increased thirst and urination
* Fatigue
* Blurred vision
* Slow-healing wounds
* Numbness or tingling in the hands or feet

Diabetes is typically diagnosed through a blood test, which measures blood sugar levels. A fasting plasma glucose (FPG) test or an oral glucose tolerance test (OGTT) may be used to diagnose diabetes.

Understanding the basics of Type 2 diabetes is the first step in managing this condition. In the following chapters, we will explore the connection between diet and Type 2 diabetes, and provide practical tips for making healthy food choices to help manage your blood sugar levels.

Chapter 2: The Connection Between Diet and Type 2 Diabetes

The food you eat plays a critical role in managing Type 2 diabetes. In this chapter, we will explore the connection between diet and Type 2 diabetes and discuss the importance of making healthy food choices.

2.1 How Diet Affects Blood Sugar Levels

The food you eat is broken down into glucose, which is then released into the bloodstream. Insulin helps to regulate the amount of glucose in the blood, but if you have Type 2 diabetes, your body becomes resistant to insulin and cannot effectively regulate blood sugar levels. This is why it's important to make healthy food choices that help to keep your blood sugar levels stable.

2.2 The Role of Nutrition in Diabetes Management

A healthy, balanced diet is essential for managing Type 2 diabetes. This includes:

* Eating plenty of fruits and vegetables

* Choosing lean sources of protein, such as chicken, fish, and tofu

* Limiting processed and sugary foods

* Incorporating healthy fats, such as avocados and nuts, into your diet

* Eating regular meals and snacks to keep your blood sugar levels stable

2.3 Practical Tips for Making Healthy Food Choices

Making healthy food choices can be challenging, especially if you're new to managing Type 2 diabetes. Here are some practical tips to help you get started:

* Keep a food diary to track your intake and identify areas for improvement

* Plan meals and snacks in advance to avoid last-minute unhealthy choices

* Read food labels to make informed decisions about what you're eating

* Eat mindfully, focusing on the taste, texture, and smell of your food

* Seek support from a registered dietitian or certified diabetes educator

By understanding the connection between diet and Type 2 diabetes, you can take control of your health and make informed decisions about the food you eat. In the following chapters, we will provide more detailed guidance on specific aspects of a healthy diet for Type 2 diabetes management.

Chapter 3: Carbohydrate Counting: A Powerful Tool for Diabetes Management

Carbohydrate counting is a key tool for managing Type 2 diabetes. In this chapter, we will explore what carbohydrate counting is, how it works, and why it's important.

3.1 What is Carbohydrate Counting?

Carbohydrate counting is a method of tracking the amount of carbohydrates you consume in a day. Carbohydrates are a type of macronutrient that is found in a wide variety of foods, including grains, fruits, vegetables, and dairy products.

3.2 How Carbohydrate Counting Works

To count carbohydrates, you will need to:

* Determine the total number of carbohydrates in a serving of food

* Add up the total number of carbohydrates you consume at each meal and snack

* Adjust your insulin dose based on your carbohydrate intake

3.3 Why Carbohydrate Counting is Important

Carbohydrate counting is important for managing Type 2 diabetes because it allows you to:

* Keep your blood sugar levels stable

* Prevent high and low blood sugar levels

* Make informed decisions about what you're eating

* Adjust your insulin dose as needed

By incorporating carbohydrate counting into your diabetes management plan, you can take control of your blood sugar levels and improve your overall health.

Chapter 4: Fiber-Rich Foods: The Secret Weapon Against Type 2 Diabetes

Fiber is an important nutrient for managing Type 2 diabetes. In this chapter, we will explore the benefits of fibre, how much fibre you need, and the best sources of fibre.

4.1 The Benefits of Fiber

Fiber has many benefits for people with Type 2 diabetes:

* Helps to slow down the absorption of glucose, preventing spikes in blood sugar levels
* Promotes feelings of fullness and satisfaction, helping to manage weight
* Supports healthy digestion and regularity
* Helps to lower cholesterol levels

4.2 How Much Fiber Do You Need?

The recommended daily intake of fibre for adults is:

* Women: 21-25 grams per day
* Men: 30-38 grams per day

4.3 The Best Sources of Fiber

The best sources of fibre include:

* Whole grains, such as brown rice, quinoa, and whole wheat bread

* Fruits and vegetables, such as berries, apples, broccoli, and Brussels sprouts

* Nuts and seeds, such as almonds, chia seeds, and flaxseeds

* Legumes, such as chickpeas, lentils, and black beans

By incorporating more fibre-rich foods into your diet, you can help to manage your blood sugar levels, support healthy digestion, and improve your overall health.

Chapter 5: Lean Proteins and Type 2 Diabetes: Choosing the Right Sources

Protein is an important nutrient for managing Type 2 diabetes, but not all protein sources are created equal. In this chapter, we will explore the benefits of lean protein, the best sources of lean protein, and how to incorporate them into your diet.

5.1 The Benefits of Lean Protein

Lean protein has many benefits for people with Type 2 diabetes:

* Helps to build and repair tissues
* Supports healthy blood sugar levels
* Promotes feelings of fullness and satisfaction
* Helps to maintain muscle mass

5.2 The Best Sources of Lean Protein

The best sources of lean protein include:

* Chicken and turkey breast
* Fish, such as salmon, tuna, and cod
* Eggs
* Tofu and other soy products
* Greek yogurt and cottage cheese
* Nuts and seeds

5.3 How to Incorporate Lean Protein into Your Diet

Here are some practical tips for incorporating lean protein into your diet:

* Choose lean cuts of meat and trim off any visible fat

* Grill, bake, or broil your protein instead of frying it

* Incorporate protein into every meal and snack

* Try new recipes and experiment with different protein sources

By choosing the right sources of lean protein, you can help to manage your blood sugar levels, support healthy digestion, and improve your overall health.

Chapter 6: Embracing Healthy Fats for Optimal Blood Sugar Control

Healthy fats are an important part of a balanced diet for people with Type 2 diabetes. In this chapter, we will explore the benefits of healthy fats, the best sources of healthy fats, and how to incorporate them into your diet.

6.1 The Benefits of Healthy Fats

Healthy fats have many benefits for people with Type 2 diabetes:

* Supports healthy blood sugar levels

* Promotes feelings of fullness and satisfaction

* Helps to reduce inflammation

* Supports healthy cholesterol levels

6.2 The Best Sources of Healthy Fats

The best sources of healthy fats include:

* Avocados

* Nuts and seeds, such as almonds, walnuts, and chia seeds

* Olive oil and other plant-based oils

* Fatty fish, such as salmon and mackerel

* Full-fat dairy products, such as Greek yogurt and cheese

6.3 How to Incorporate Healthy Fats into Your Diet

Here are some practical tips for incorporating healthy fats into your diet:

* Use olive oil or avocado oil for cooking and baking

* Top your salads and vegetables with nuts and seeds

* Incorporate avocado into your meals and snacks

* Choose full-fat dairy products instead of low-fat or fat-free options

By embracing healthy fats, you can help to manage your blood sugar levels, support healthy digestion, and improve your overall health.

Chapter 7: The Dark Side of Added Sugars: How to Limit Your Intake

Added sugars can wreak havoc on blood sugar levels for people with Type 2 diabetes. In this chapter, we will explore the dangers of added sugars, how to identify added sugars, and how to limit your intake.

7.1 The Dangers of Added Sugars

Added sugars can:

* Cause spikes in blood sugar levels

* Lead to weight gain

* Increase the risk of heart disease

* Increase the risk of dental cavities

7.2 How to Identify Added Sugars

Added sugars can be found in a wide variety of foods, including:

* Sugary drinks, such as soda, sweet tea, and sports drinks

* Candy and other sweets

* Baked goods, such as cakes, cookies, and pastries

* Processed foods, such as frozen meals, canned soups, and granola bars

To identify added sugars, look for the following ingredients on food labels:

* Sugar

* High fructose corn syrup

* Brown sugar

* Corn syrup

* Dextrose

* Fructose

* Glucose

* Honey

* Maple syrup

* Molasses

* Sucrose

7.3 How to Limit Your Intake of Added Sugars

Here are some practical tips for limiting your intake of added sugars:

* Choose water or unsweetened tea instead of sugary drinks

* Limit your intake of candy and other sweets

* Choose whole, unprocessed foods instead of processed foods

* Read food labels and choose products with the least amount of added sugars

* Try natural sweeteners, such as stevia or erythritol, instead of sugar

By limiting your intake of added sugars, you can help to manage your blood sugar levels, support healthy digestion, and improve your overall health.

[Continuation confirmation received?] [Continue to Chapter 8]

Chapter 8: Mastering Meal Planning and Portion Control

Meal planning and portion control are essential for managing Type 2 diabetes. In this chapter, we will explore the benefits of meal planning and portion control, and provide practical tips for mastering these skills.

8.1 The Benefits of Meal Planning and Portion Control

Meal planning and portion control have many benefits for people with Type 2 diabetes:

* Helps to keep blood sugar levels stable

* Supports healthy digestion

* Promotes weight management

* Reduces the risk of overeating

8.2 Practical Tips for Meal Planning

Here are some practical tips for meal planning:

* Plan your meals and snacks for the week ahead

* Choose a variety of whole, unprocessed foods

* Incorporate lean protein, fibre-rich fruits and vegetables, and healthy fats into each meal

* Prepare meals in advance to save time during the week

* Use meal planning apps or tools to make the process easier

8.3 Practical Tips for Portion Control

Here are some practical tips for portion control:

* Use smaller plates and bowls to help control portion sizes
* Measure out your food to ensure accurate portion sizes
* Eat slowly and mindfully
* Listen to your body's hunger and fullness cues
* Avoid distractions, such as watching TV or working, while eating

By mastering meal planning and portion control, you can take control of your blood sugar levels, support healthy digestion, and improve your overall health.

Chapter 9: Common Misconceptions About Diabetes and Diet: Separating Fact from Fiction

There are many misconceptions about diabetes and diet. In this chapter, we will explore some of the most common misconceptions and separate fact from fiction.

9.1 Misconception: People with Diabetes Cannot Eat Sugar

Fact: People with diabetes can eat sugar, but they should limit their intake and choose natural sources of sugar, such as fruit, instead of added sugars.

9.2 Misconception: People with Diabetes Need to Eat Specially-Marketed Diabetes Products

Fact: People with diabetes do not need to eat specially-marketed diabetes products. Instead, they should focus on eating whole, unprocessed foods.

9.3 Misconception: People with Diabetes Cannot Eat Carbohydrates

Fact: People with diabetes can eat carbohydrates, but they should choose complex carbohydrates, such as whole grains and vegetables, instead of simple carbohydrates, such as white bread and sugary drinks.

Chapter 10: Monitoring Blood Sugar Levels: The Key to Effective Diabetes Management

Monitoring blood sugar levels is an essential part of effective diabetes management. In this chapter, we will explore the importance of monitoring blood sugar levels, how to monitor your blood sugar levels, and what to do if your blood sugar levels are out of range.

10.1 The Importance of Monitoring Blood Sugar Levels

Monitoring blood sugar levels can help you:

* Keep your blood sugar levels stable

* Prevent high and low blood sugar levels

* Make informed decisions about your diet and lifestyle

* Detect and prevent complications

10.2 How to Monitor Your Blood Sugar Levels

To monitor your blood sugar levels, you will need a blood glucose meter and test strips. Follow these steps to test your blood sugar levels:

* Wash your hands with soap and warm water

* Insert a test strip into the meter

* Prick your finger with a lancet

* Place a drop of blood on the test strip

* Wait for the meter to display your blood sugar level

10.3 What to Do if Your Blood Sugar Levels Are Out of Range

If your blood sugar levels are out of range, take the following steps:

* Check your blood sugar levels again to confirm the reading

* If your blood sugar levels are too high, take your prescribed medication and make adjustments to your diet and lifestyle

* If your blood sugar levels are too low, consume 15-20 grams of fast-acting carbohydrates, such as fruit juice or glucose tablets

By monitoring your blood sugar levels, you can take control of your diabetes management and improve your overall health.

Exercise is a powerful tool for managing Type 2 diabetes. In this chapter, we will explore the benefits of exercise, the best types of exercise for people with Type 2 diabetes, and how to get started with an exercise routine.

11.1 The Benefits of Exercise

Exercise has many benefits for people with Type 2 diabetes:

* Helps to lower blood sugar levels

* Promotes weight loss

* Supports healthy digestion

* Improves cardiovascular health

* Boosts energy levels

11.2 The Best Types of Exercise

The best types of exercise for people with Type 2 diabetes include:

* Aerobic exercise, such as walking, cycling, and swimming

* Resistance training, such as weight lifting and bodyweight exercises

* Flexibility exercises, such as yoga and tai chi

11.3 How to Get Started with an Exercise Routine

Here are some practical tips for getting started with an exercise routine:

* Consult with your healthcare provider before starting an exercise routine

* Start slowly and gradually increase the intensity and duration of your workouts

* Choose activities that you enjoy

* Set realistic goals

* Find a workout buddy or join a fitness class for support and motivation

By incorporating exercise into your diabetes management plan, you can take control of your blood sugar levels, support healthy digestion, and improve your overall health.

Chapter 12: Emotional Well-Being and Type 2 Diabetes Management: A Holistic Approach

Managing Type 2 diabetes is not just about diet and exercise. Emotional well-being also plays a critical role in effective diabetes management. In this chapter, we will explore the importance of emotional well-being, common emotional challenges faced by people with Type 2 diabetes, and practical tips for managing emotional well-being.

12.1 The Importance of Emotional Well-Being

Emotional well-being is important for overall health and well-being, and it plays a critical role in effective diabetes management. When you feel emotionally well, you are better able to manage your diabetes and make healthy choices.

12.2 Common Emotional Challenges

People with Type 2 diabetes may face a variety of emotional challenges, including:

* Stress

* Anxiety

* Depression

* Burnout

* Grief and loss

12.3 Practical Tips for Managing Emotional Well-Being

Here are some practical tips for managing emotional well-being:

* Practice stress management techniques, such as deep breathing and meditation
* Seek support from family, friends, and healthcare professionals
* Join a support group for people with Type 2 diabetes
* Engage in activities that bring you joy and fulfilment
* Prioritize self-care, such as getting enough sleep and taking breaks throughout the day

By prioritizing emotional well-being, you can take control of your diabetes management and improve your overall health.

Chapter 13: Support and Resources for Type 2 Diabetes Management

Managing Type 2 diabetes can be challenging, but there are many supports and resources available to help. In this chapter, we will explore some of the most helpful support and resources for people with Type 2 diabetes.

13.1 Healthcare Professionals

Here are some examples of healthcare professionals that can be important for people with Type 2 diabetes:

* Endocrinologists: Endocrinologists are specialists in hormonal disorders, including diabetes. They can provide expert care and guidance for managing Type 2 diabetes, including medication management, lifestyle changes, and monitoring blood sugar levels.

* Dietitians: Registered dietitians can provide valuable guidance on dietary changes for managing Type 2 diabetes. They can help individuals develop a healthy, balanced eating plan that meets their individual needs and preferences, while also supporting blood sugar control.

* Certified Diabetes Educators (CDEs): CDEs are healthcare professionals who have special training and expertise in diabetes education. They can provide education and support on a wide range of topics related to diabetes management, including medication, diet, exercise, and monitoring blood sugar levels.

* Primary Care Physicians: Primary care physicians, such as family doctors or internists, can provide basic care and guidance for managing Type 2 diabetes. They can monitor blood sugar levels, prescribe medication, and provide referrals to specialists as needed.

* Nurse Practitioners and Physician Assistants: Nurse practitioners and physician assistants can provide basic care and guidance for managing Type 2 diabetes under the supervision of a physician. They can monitor blood sugar levels, prescribe medication, and provide education on diabetes management.

* Podiatrists: Podiatrists are foot specialists who can provide care and guidance for preventing and treating foot problems, which are a common complication of diabetes.

* Eye Doctors: Eye doctors, such as ophthalmologists or optometrists, can provide regular eye exams to monitor for diabetes-related eye problems, such as diabetic retinopathy.

* Mental Health Professionals: Mental health professionals, such as therapists or counsellors, can provide support for managing the emotional challenges of living with Type 2 diabetes. They can help individuals develop coping skills, manage stress, and improve their overall well-being.

By working with a team of healthcare professionals, people with Type 2 diabetes can receive comprehensive care and support for managing their condition and improving their overall health.

13.2 Support Groups

Diabetes support groups can be an invaluable resource for individuals with Type 2 diabetes. These groups provide a safe and supportive environment where individuals can share their experiences, ask questions, and learn from others who are going through similar challenges.

There are several types of diabetes support groups, including:

* In-person support groups: These groups meet in person at a designated location, such as a community centre or healthcare facil-

ity. They are typically led by a healthcare professional or a trained volunteer.

* Online support groups: Online support groups provide a virtual space for individuals with Type 2 diabetes to connect and share their experiences. These groups may be hosted on social media platforms, message boards, or dedicated websites.

* Peer support programs: Peer support programs connect individuals with Type 2 diabetes with trained peer mentors who have lived experience managing the condition. These mentors can provide guidance, support, and encouragement, and help individuals develop coping skills and strategies for managing their diabetes.

* Family and friends support groups: These groups provide education and support for the family members and friends of individuals with Type 2 diabetes. They can help loved ones better understand the condition, learn how to provide support, and develop coping strategies for their own emotional well-being.

Participating in a diabetes support group can provide many benefits, including:

* Improved knowledge and understanding of diabetes management

* Increased confidence and self-efficacy

* Improved emotional well-being and reduced stress

* A sense of connection and community

* Access to valuable resources and information

When choosing a diabetes support group, it's important to consider factors such as the group's size, format, and leadership. It may also be helpful to attend a few different groups to find one that feels like a good fit.

Overall, diabetes support groups can be a valuable resource for individuals with Type 2 diabetes, providing education, support, and a sense of community to help them manage their condition and improve their overall health.

13.3 Educational Resources

Books:

There are many books available that provide valuable information and insights on managing Type 2 diabetes. Some popular options include "The Diabetes Code" by Dr. Jason Fung, "The Blood Sugar Solution" by Dr. Mark Hyman, and "The Complete Diabetes Cookbook" by the American Diabetes Association.

Websites:

There are many websites that offer free resources and information on managing Type 2 diabetes. Some reputable options include the American Diabetes Association (www.diabetes.org), the National Institute of Diabetes and Digestive and Kidney Diseases (www.niddk.nih.gov), and the Mayo Clinic (www.mayoclinic.org).

Podcasts:

Podcasts can be a great way to learn about managing Type 2 diabetes while on the go. Some popular diabetes podcasts include "The Diabetes Daily Grind," "The Diabetes Power Show," and "The Diabetes Connections Podcast."

Online Communities: Joining online communities, such as forums or social media groups, can provide a sense of connection and support for people with Type 2 diabetes. These communities can be a great place to ask questions, share experiences, and learn from others.

Educational Programs:

Many healthcare organizations and community centres offer educational programs for people with Type 2 diabetes. These programs can provide valuable information and support for managing diabetes, as well as the opportunity to connect with others who are going through similar experiences.

By taking advantage of these educational resources, people with Type 2 diabetes can empower themselves with knowledge and make informed decisions about their diabetes management.

13.4 Medical Devices

There are a variety of medical devices available to help individuals with Type 2 diabetes manage their condition. Here are some examples:

1. Blood glucose meters: These devices measure blood glucose levels by analysing a small drop of blood. They are portable and easy to use, and can provide quick and accurate results.

2. Continuous glucose monitors (CGMs): CGMs are small devices that are worn on the body and measure glucose levels continuously throughout the day and night. They can provide real-time data and alerts for high or low glucose levels, and can help individuals better understand their glucose patterns and make more informed decisions about their diabetes management.

3. Insulin pumps: Insulin pumps are small devices that deliver insulin continuously through a catheter placed under the skin. They can be programmed to deliver insulin based on an individual's needs, and can help improve glucose control and reduce the risk of hypoglycaemia.

4. Smart insulin pens: Smart insulin pens are insulin pens that track insulin doses and provide data on insulin use. They can help individuals manage their insulin doses more effectively and improve their overall diabetes management.

5. Automated insulin delivery systems: Automated insulin deliv-

ery systems, also known as artificial pancreas systems, are systems that automatically adjust insulin delivery based on real-time glucose data. They can help improve glucose control and reduce the risk of hypoglycaemia.

6. Diabetes management apps: Diabetes management apps can help individuals track their blood glucose levels, medications, meals, and physical activity. They can provide reminders and alerts, and can help individuals better understand their diabetes management and make more informed decisions.

When choosing a medical device for Type 2 diabetes management, it's important to consider factors such as ease of use, accuracy, cost, and compatibility with other devices or systems. It may also be helpful to consult with a healthcare professional to determine the most appropriate device for an individual's needs.

Medical devices can be a valuable tool for managing Type 2 diabetes, providing real-time data and alerts, improving glucose control, and reducing the risk of complications. By working with a healthcare professional and choosing the right device, individuals with Type 2 diabetes can take an active role in managing their condition and improving their overall health.

Chapter 14: Empowering Yourself: The Path to a Healthy, Fulfilling Life

Empowering yourself is an essential step in managing Type 2 diabetes and living a healthy, fulfilling life. Here are some strategies for empowering yourself and taking control of your diabetes management:

1. Take charge of your healthcare: This means being proactive in your diabetes management, asking questions, and seeking out information about your condition. It also means working closely with your healthcare team and making informed decisions about your care.

2. Set goals: Setting specific, measurable, and achievable goals for your diabetes management can help you stay motivated and on track. These goals might include improving your blood glucose control, increasing your physical activity, or making healthy dietary changes.

3. Seek support: Having a strong support system can make a big difference in your diabetes management. Seek out support from family, friends, and healthcare professionals, and consider joining a diabetes support group to connect with others who are going through similar challenges.

4. Stay informed: Keeping up-to-date with the latest research and developments in Type 2 diabetes management can help you make informed decisions about your care. Consider subscribing to diabetes-related newsletters or following reputable diabetes organizations on social media.

5. Practice self-care: Taking care of yourself, both physically and emotionally, is essential for effective diabetes management. This might include engaging in regular physical activity, getting enough sleep, managing stress, and making time for activities that bring you joy and fulfilment.

6. Seek out resources: There are many resources available to help individuals with Type 2 diabetes manage their condition. These might include diabetes education programs, online resources, or mobile apps. Take advantage of these resources to help you stay on track with your diabetes management.

By empowering yourself and taking an active role in your diabetes management, you can improve your blood glucose control, reduce your risk of complications, and live a healthy, fulfilling life. Remember, you are the expert in your own diabetes management, and by working closely with your healthcare team and seeking out support and resources, you can achieve your goals and thrive.

14.1 The Importance of Empowerment

Empowerment is an essential component of effective Type 2 diabetes management. When individuals with Type 2 diabetes feel empowered, they are better able to take an active role in managing their condition and making informed decisions about their healthcare.

Empowerment can take many forms, including:

1. Knowledge: Gaining knowledge about Type 2 diabetes, including its causes, symptoms, and treatment options, can help individuals feel more confident and in control of their condition.

2. Skills: Developing skills in areas such as meal planning, physical activity, and blood glucose monitoring can help individuals with Type 2 diabetes manage their condition more effectively and improve their overall health.

3. Support: Having a strong support system, including family, friends, and healthcare professionals, can help individuals with Type 2 diabetes feel more empowered and confident in their ability to manage their condition.

4. Autonomy: Feeling in control of their diabetes management and having the ability to make decisions about their care can help individuals with Type 2 diabetes feel more empowered and engaged in their healthcare.

5. Resilience: Developing resilience and coping skills can help individuals with Type 2 diabetes navigate the challenges of living with a chronic condition and maintain a positive outlook.

When individuals with Type 2 diabetes feel empowered, they are more likely to take an active role in managing their condition, adhere to treatment recommendations, and achieve better health outcomes.

Empowerment can be fostered through a variety of strategies, including:

1. Education: Providing individuals with Type 2 diabetes with accurate and relevant information about their condition can help them feel more knowledgeable and empowered.

2. Skill-building: Teaching individuals with Type 2 diabetes skills in areas such as meal planning, physical activity, and blood glucose monitoring can help them feel more confident and capable in managing their condition.

3. Support: Providing individuals with Type 2 diabetes with a strong support system, including family, friends, and healthcare professionals, can help them feel more empowered and engaged in their healthcare.

4. Collaboration: Encouraging collaboration between individuals with Type 2 diabetes and their healthcare professionals can help foster a sense of autonomy and empowerment.

5. Resilience-building: Teaching individuals with Type 2 diabetes resilience and coping skills can help them navigate the challenges of living with a chronic condition and maintain a positive outlook.

By fostering empowerment, individuals with Type 2 diabetes can take an active role in managing their condition, make informed decisions about their healthcare, and achieve better health outcomes.

14.2 The Benefits of Taking Control of Your Diabetes Management

Taking control of your diabetes management can have many benefits, including:

* Improved blood sugar control

* Better overall health

* Increased energy and vitality

* A sense of accomplishment and empowerment

14.3 Practical Tips for Empowering Yourself

Here are some practical tips for empowering yourself:

* Set realistic goals and celebrate your successes

* Take an active role in your diabetes management

* Seek support from family, friends, and healthcare professionals

* Educate yourself about diabetes and its management

* Be kind and compassionate with yourself

By empowering yourself, you can take control of your diabetes management, improve your overall health, and live a healthy, fulfilling life.